Ready-Set-PN
Preparing for the NCLEX-PN®

Editors

Assessment Technologies Institute®, LLC, Curriculum Team

Associate Editor

Brant Stacy, BS Journalism, BA English
Product Developer

COPYRIGHT NOTICE

D1418265

Table of Contents

Table of Contents

Preparing for the NCLEX-PN®

- Whether you have always wanted to be a nurse or nursing is not your first career choice, you have been working diligently for some time in a nursing program. However, once you graduate, you still have to pass the NCLEX-PN. This booklet will introduce you to some information, techniques, and tips you'll surely find helpful as you prepare for this licensure examination.

- Join us as ATI helps you get ready... set... be a practical nurse!

- To ensure public safety, regulatory agencies within each U.S. state and territory control the granting of licensure to practice as a registered nurse (RN) or a licensed practical/vocational nurse (PN). The National Council of State Boards of Nursing (NCSBN) develops and administers the two licensing examinations (RN and PN) these regulatory agencies use to make licensing decisions. To practice as an PN, you must pass the National Council Licensure Examination for Practical/Vocational Nurses (NCLEX-PN). This examination measures your ability to be a safe, effective, entry-level PN.

- Contributing to the development and administration of the NCLEX are the examination committee, the item review subcommittee, the NCSBN NCLEX staff, and Pearson VUE test services.

Information About the NCLEX-PN

- The NCLEX-PN test plan is revised every 3 years. The current test plan, available at www.ncsbn.org, lists the major categories and nursing activities that guide the test's content. You'll find the most comprehensive information about registering for the NCLEX-PN in the candidate bulletin, also available at www.ncsbn.org. A new bulletin is published each January.

- The NCLEX-PN Registration Process

  ○ Submit an application for licensure to the board of nursing in the state where you want to be licensed. Each state has a process for approving candidates for licensure and determining eligibility for testing. Be sure to follow your school's protocol to prevent delays in processing.

  ○ Meet all requirements of your state's board of nursing. When your board determines that you are eligible, it will send that information to the NCSBN.

  ○ Register with Pearson VUE either through the Internet or by mail.

    ■ Internet registration may be completed at www.pearsonvue.com/nclex (select the "Create an Account and register" link).

    ■ Registration may be sent through the U.S. Postal Service. The registration form must be mailed along with a certified check, cashier's check, or money order for $200 (made payable to the National Council of State Boards of Nursing) to: NCLEX Operations, PO Box 64950, St. Paul, MN 55164-0950.

- Apply to Pearson VUE to take the NCLEX-PN when you apply to your state's board of nursing so that Pearson VUE will already have your information when it receives your approval to test. You should have a confirmation of receipt of your application within 2 weeks. When your board forwards the approval to test to the NCSBN, Pearson VUE will send you an authorization to test (ATT). The ATT will contain your test authorization number, your candidate identification number, and an expiration date. Your board will determine how long the ATT is valid; this varies from state to state between 60 and 395 days, with an average of 90 days. You may test only within this time period. It cannot be extended for any reason.

- Schedule your test date as soon as possible after receiving your ATT. This does not mean you need to test immediately, but test centers fill up rapidly and it may be difficult to arrange the date you want. In addition, if you wait too long, there might be no dates left within your valid testing time. First-time candidates receive a test date within 30 days of their telephone request and repeat test takers within 45 days, but you may decline and request a later date. To schedule your test, call NCLEX Candidate Services or go to www.pearsonvue.com/nclex.

About Scheduling the Test

- Be realistic when scheduling your test appointment, allowing at least a month to transition from school to preparing for the test. Avoid time periods that might be stressful for you. While preparing, review course materials and class notes, practice as many questions as you can, and then test. Waiting more than 5 months can erode your confidence and distract you from your purpose. Schedule the test within a reasonable time frame to maximize your chances of success.

- Go to www.pearsonvue.com/nclex to find testing center locations. Identify several possibilities and their ease of access from your home so that you have more than one option. You may test in any city or state; the testing center is not linked to your state of initial licensure. Make a list of potential sites, dates, and your preferred time of day and have it ready when you call.

Develop a Study Plan With a Readiness Target

- Plan to set a target of 1 week before the test for reaching your study goals. Use your results from ATI comprehensive assessments and predictors to identify the content areas you need to study. Be sure to access the focused review soon after completing each ATI assessment. Use your class notes and all your ATI materials and programs to help you review. Setting manageable goals for each component of your study plan will make it easier to complete it by your target date. If you enroll in Virtual ATI®, your instructor will help you make a plan and set a date.

Review Your Examinations

- When faculty offer you a test review session before or after tests, take advantage of these opportunities. Review sessions before tests will help you focus your study efforts. Review sessions after examinations will help you obtain more information about missed items so that you can improve your understanding of the content.

Use Your Achievement Tests

- Faculty select standardized achievement tests to help you prepare for the NCLEX-PN and can help you interpret test scores. These tests validate your application of knowledge and guide you toward areas to study. Doing your best on achievement tests can boost your confidence as you approach the NCLEX-PN. Use your results to improve your test-taking skills and to focus on specific content areas. Take your achievement tests seriously and participate in reviewing the results.

Read Your Textbooks

- How can you best use the resources your faculty provides? Read the assignments prior to class. After class, go back to the textbooks and reread the tables, look at the figures and diagrams, discuss the care plans and maps, and respond to the critical-thinking questions and clinical scenarios. This will help you focus on relevant information that will support your NCLEX-PN preparation. When studying for remediation, study the related review modules and go back to the textbooks to read the content again.

Complete the NCLEX-PN Tutorial

- Go to www.pearsonvue.com/nclex, scroll down to the online tutorial, and click on it. Even though you'll view this tutorial on your test day, the more familiar you become with the NCLEX-PN screens and processes, the easier the test can seem. Practice using the calculator on the computer.

Stay Healthy

- Do what keeps you healthy and fit. Exercise, eat healthful and balanced meals and snacks, stay hydrated, read, practice relaxation techniques, and visit with family and friends. If you usually drink caffeinated beverages, have a light or moderate amount prior to the test. Don't overdo it to the point where caffeine affects your performance. Be sure to get adequate rest the night before the test.

Your Work Schedule

- Discuss your test date with your employer. If possible, request time off the week before the test to make sure you are well rested.

Changing or Canceling Your Appointment

- If you choose to change your appointment, you must do this at least one full business day before your test time. For example, if your test is at 10:00 a.m. on Monday, you must change it by 10:00 a.m. the Friday before. There is no charge for this change, but you will forfeit the test fee if you make any changes after that point. You must then reschedule online at www.pearsonvue.com/nclex or by phone. If you do not arrive on time, you also forfeit your time slot and test fee, and you must register and pay again.

- Cancel your test appointment only after considering all options and making the best possible decision. Regardless of the reason, you will forfeit the test fee and must reapply and pay again.

Finding the Testing Center

- Use a map search engine on the Internet to check the directions to the address of your testing location. Be sure you know exactly where you are going ahead of time and allow enough time to arrive 30 min before your test time whether you are driving or taking public transportation. If you are at all unsure, consider driving there or taking public transportation a few days beforehand to confirm your route.

What to Bring to the Testing Center

- You must bring your valid ATT and one form of acceptable photo identification with a signature, such as a U.S. driver's license or a passport. Without these materials, you won't be permitted to test and will forfeit the test fee. You'll have to reschedule and pay again. Testing center staff will take your fingerprint and photo and ask you to provide your signature. Pearson VUE also uses palm-vein technology at test centers as a secondary measure of security.

- You may not bring any study materials into the testing facility. You'll have a small locker for storing your personal items. You must turn off your cell phone and/or pager and store them in the locker, along with all electronic devices, bags, purses, backpacks, coats, hats, food, beverages, gum, lip balm, and other items detailed in the candidate bulletin. You may use only the calculator on the computer.

About the Test

- The NCLEX-PN uses computerized adaptive testing (CAT), a system that will select test items for you based on your ability to answer previous items. In other words, each time you answer a question, CAT determines the next question based on its estimate that you will have a 50% chance of answering the question correctly. That way, your next question will not be too easy or too difficult, and how you answer gives CAT good information about your overall ability to pass the test. By targeting the test items specifically for you, CAT can generate your test results by using fewer items than would be required with standard "percentage correct" testing.

- You must answer a minimum of 85 questions but possibly up to 205 questions. The test will end when CAT determines with 95% certainty that your ability is either below or above the passing standard, the maximum amount of time has elapsed, or you have answered the maximum number of questions.

- You will have 5 hr to complete the test. There will be two optional breaks, one after 2 hr and another after 3½ hr. If you feel you need a break, it may be to your advantage to take one. Time away from the test may help you feel more refreshed and ready to continue. It is important to remember, however, that break time is part of the 5 hr.

- Although there is no time limit per question, it is important to keep a steady pace when testing. Try not to spend more than 2 min on each item, as the test will not progress if you do not select an answer for each question. But do not make rapid guesses, either, as it can work against you with CAT. Read each item carefully, consider the options, make your selection, and move to the next item. You cannot go back to any previous questions.

Confidentiality

- Disclosing test items before, during, or after the examination is a violation of law. This means that posting, sharing, or discussing items that you remember could result in legal and/or disciplinary action.

Getting Your Results

- Visit the Web site of your state's board of nursing to find out how to obtain your test results. All states will provide written notification of your results with appropriate documentation by ground mail. You may also access a "quick results" service for an unofficial report at www.pearsonvue.com/nclex. If you do not pass the test, you may retest after the waiting period your board requires.

The Test Plan for the NCLEX-PN

- The NCLEX-PN is constructed according to a test plan that outlines the content of the test questions, with client needs as the test's framework. The scope of content is based on data from the most recent practice analysis (2009) – the results of a survey of 150 tasks and responsibilities of newly licensed PNs in the U.S. The examination includes application-based scenarios in the clinical areas of medical-surgical, maternal newborn, mental health, and nursing care of children. It integrates into all client need categories several additional concepts and processes fundamental to safe and effective practice at the entry level, including caring, communication, documentation, the nursing process, teaching, and learning.

Client Need Categories

- The NCLEX-PN's test plan is organized according to client needs, a concept that provides a structure for nursing actions and competencies across all settings for all clients. The NCLEX-PN has predetermined percentages of test items for each client need category or subcategory, as follows:
- Safe and Effective Care Environment
  - Coordinated Care – 13% to 19%
  - Safety and Infection Control – 11% to 17%
- Health Promotion and Maintenance – 7% to 13%
- Psychosocial Integrity – 7% to 13%

- Physiological Integrity
  - Basic Care and Comfort – 9% to 15%
  - Pharmacological and Parenteral Therapies – 11% to 17%
  - Reduction of Risk Potential – 9% to 15%
  - Physiological Adaptation – 9% to 15%
- Most test items address the application level of cognitive ability (requiring more complex thought processing) or higher. The NCLEX-PN's reading level does not exceed 10th grade. Its intent is not to test your ability to read, but to determine your level of proficiency in understanding nursing concepts and activities.
- The tables on the following pages outline how the NCLEX-PN test plan incorporates the four major categories of client needs. These lists present examples of the types of test content and topics, but they are not all-inclusive. For lists of the actual activity statements and tasks on which the items are based, access the "Test Plans" menu selection at www.ncsbn.org.

CLIENT NEED:
Safe and Effective Care Environment

Coordinated Care 13% to 19%	Examples of Test Content
	• Advance directives
	• Advocacy
	• Client care assignments
	• Clients' rights
	• Collaboration with the interdisciplinary team
	• Concepts of management and supervision
	• Confidentiality and information security
	• Continuity of care
	• Establishment of priorities
	• Ethical practice
	• Information technology
	• Informed consent
	• Legal rights and responsibilities
	• Performance and quality improvement
	• Referrals
	• Resource management

Safe and Effective Care Environment
Examples of Test Topics

- Accessing clients' records using facility regulations
- Advocating for clients
- Assigning client care delivery
- Assisting new employees during orientation
- Collaborating with the interdisciplinary team when providing care
- Collecting data and prioritizing care for an assigned group of clients
- Documenting clients' data using computerized formats
- Ensuring client's confidentiality and privacy
- Following the chain of command when assisting with the resolution of staff conflicts
- Following up with clients and families after discharge
- Making clinical decisions using data from various sources
- Participating in quality improvement activities
- Participating in the development of care plans
- Participating in the informed consent process
- Participating in transcribing verbal and telephone prescriptions
- Performing telephone triage
- Promoting clients' involvement in decision making
- Proving input into the performance evaluations of other staff
- Reinforcing teaching to clients and families about advance directives
- Reporting a provider's unsafe practice activities (improper care, substance abuse)
- Reporting issues such as abuse and communicable disease per facility policies
- Seeking assistance when unable to perform assigned tasks
- Transferring and discharging clients according to facility policies
- Using information technology in various health care settings
- Using research when providing care

CLIENT NEED:		
Safe and Effective Care Environment		
Safety and Infection Control 11% to 17%	Examples of Test Content	
	• Accident and injury prevention • Emergency response plans • Ergonomic principles • Error prevention • Handling hazardous and infectious materials • Home safety • Reports of incidents, events ,irregular occurrences, and variances • Safe use of equipment • Security plans • Standard and transmission-based precautions and surgical asepsis • Use of restraints and safety devices	
Examples of Test Topics		

- Adhering to procedures for handling biohazardous materials
- Applying restraints safely and using the least restrictive devices
- Checking the accuracy of treatment prescriptions
- Collecting data about and documenting clients' allergies
- Contributing to and implementing internal and external disaster plans
- Implementing monitoring procedures (restraint checks, seizure precautions)
- Maintaining medical and surgical asepsis
- Operating and maintaining equipment safely
- Preparing a variance or incident report
- Providing care using ergonomic principles
- Providing information to clients and families about home safety
- Reinforcing teaching to clients and staff about infection control
- Reinforcing teaching to clients and staff about injury prevention
- Using triage and evacuation protocols
- Verifying clients' identity

CLIENT NEED:		
Health Promotion and Maintenance		
Health Promotion and Maintenance 7 to 13%	Examples of Test Content	
	• Aging process • Ante/intra/postpartum and newborn care • Data collection techniques • Developmental stages and transitions • Health promotion and disease prevention • High-risk behaviors • Lifestyle choices • Self-care	
Examples of Test Topics		

- Assisting clients with family-planning needs
- Caring for clients prenatally
- Choosing developmentally appropriate nursing interventions for clients of various ages
- Collecting data from clients
- Determining clients' abilities to perform self-care activities
- Monitoring clients in labor
- Promoting participation in health screening programs
- Providing care to clients after delivery
- Providing information to clients about high-risk behaviors
- Providing newborn care and nutrition information
- Reinforcing teaching about immunization schedules
- Reinforcing teaching about self-examination screening techniques

CLIENT NEED:	
Psychosocial Integrity	
Psychosocial Integrity 7 to 13%	**Examples of Test Content** • Abuse and neglect • Behavioral interventions • Chemical and other dependencies • Coping mechanisms • Crisis intervention • Cultural diversity • End-of-life care • Grief and loss • Mental health concepts • Religious and spiritual influences on health • Sensory and perceptual alterations • Stress management • Support systems • Therapeutic communication • Therapeutic environment

Examples of Test Topics

- Collecting data from clients suspected of chemical dependency, withdrawal, or toxicity
- Communicating with clients who are not following the treatment plan
- Determining clients' potential for violence
- Developing therapeutic relationships with clients and families
- Encouraging clients' participation in group sessions
- Examining reasons for clients' behavior
- Helping clients adjust to changes in body image to promote recovery
- Offering emotional support to clients and families
- Participating in planning and intervening for clients and families during end-of-life care
- Participating in the care of clients with non-substance-related dependencies
- Participating in various types of therapies (reminiscence, validation)
- Promoting effective coping of clients and families
- Providing a therapeutic environment to help manage behavior
- Providing care for clients and families at risk for abuse or who have been abused

Psychosocial Integrity
Examples of Test Topics

- Providing care for clients and families based on cultural beliefs about health practices
- Providing support during times of grief and loss
- Recognizing the needs of clients whose sensory perceptions are distorted
- Reinforcing teaching for caregivers of clients with mental disorders
- Reinforcing teaching for clients and families about clients' psychosocial status

CLIENT NEED:
Physiological Integrity

Basic Care and Comfort 9% to 15%	Examples of Test Content
	• Assistive devices
	• Elimination
	• Mobility and immobility
	• Nonpharmacological comfort interventions
	• Nutrition and oral hydration
	• Personal hygiene
	• Rest and sleep

Examples of Test Topics

- Administering enteral feedings safely
- Assisting clients with self-care and ADLs
- Collecting and recording intake and output data
- Encouraging clients' independence in eating
- Helping clients make appropriate dietary choices
- Helping clients meet their needs for rest and sleep
- Helping clients meet their nutritional and hydration needs
- Implementing measures to promote skin integrity and prevent pressure-related injuries
- Incorporating alternative and complementary therapies when planning care
- Keeping clients in correct body alignment
- Promoting urinary and bowel elimination
- Providing care for clients in traction or other immobilizing devices
- Providing care to maximize clients' mobility
- Providing nonpharmacological measures to relieve pain
- Using proper body mechanics and assistive devices when moving clients

CLIENT NEED:		
Physiological Integrity		
Pharmacological and Parenteral Therapies 11% to 17%	Examples of Test Content	
	• Adverse and side effects, contraindications, and interactions • Dosage calculation • Expected actions and outcomes • Medication administration • Pharmacological pain management	
Examples of Test Topics		

- Calculating medication doses
- Following facility policies for documenting medication administration
- Following regulations for administering and disposing of controlled substances
- Identifying interactions among medications
- Identifying side and adverse effects of medication therapy
- Monitoring and intervening for responses to medications
- Preparing, administering, and documenting medications
- Recognizing data to collect prior to medication administration
- Recognizing incompatibilities among prescribed medications
- Recognizing precautions and contraindications for medications
- Reinforcing teaching about how to self-administer medications
- Reviewing pharmacological agents in light of clients' pathophysiology

CLIENT NEED:		
Physiological Integrity		
Reduction of Risk Potential 9% to 15%	**Examples of Test Content**	
	• Changes and abnormalities in vital signs • Diagnostic tests • Laboratory values • Potential for alterations in body systems • Potential for complications from surgical procedures and health alterations • Possible complications of diagnostic tests, treatments, and procedures • Therapeutic procedures	
Examples of Test Topics		

- Caring for clients undergoing procedures or treatments
- Collecting clients' data (vital signs, oxygen saturation, neurological and circulatory checks)
- Collecting data about risk potential related to falls, mobility status, and sensory impairment
- Collecting specimens for diagnostic testing (blood, stool, urine, sputum)
- Inserting, maintaining the patency of, and removing tubes (NG, indwelling urinary catheter)
- Monitoring clients following an unusual occurrence (fall, medication error)
- Monitoring clients for alterations in body systems
- Monitoring the function of therapeutic devices
- Performing an electrocardiogram and intervening as directed
- Providing care and maintaining safety for clients undergoing surgery
- Providing care to clients with continuous or intermittent NG suction
- Providing preoperative and postoperative care
- Recognizing laboratory values and deviations from expected ranges

CLIENT NEED:
Physiological Integrity

Physiological Adaptation 9% to 15%	Examples of Test Content
	• Alterations in body systems • Basic pathophysiology • Fluid and electrolyte imbalances • Medical emergencies • Radiation therapy • Unexpected responses to therapies

Examples of Test Topics

- Caring for clients receiving mechanical ventilation
- Detecting cardiac monitoring abnormalities
- Giving care to clients who have complications of pregnancy, labor, and delivery
- Monitoring and documenting clients' fluid and electrolyte status
- Monitoring clients for indications of infection
- Notifying the provider of a change in clients' status
- Performing CPR
- Providing care for clients with an unexpected response to therapy
- Providing care for newborns requiring phototherapy
- Providing care to clients requiring respiratory assistance (choking, dyspnea)
- Providing care to clients who have a tracheostomy
- Providing emergency care for clients who have injuries or have had trauma
- Providing wound care, including the removal of wound sutures or staples
- Reinforcing teaching for clients after radiation therapy

TEST-TAKING STRATEGIES

Reading Test Items

- The amount of information in a test item can overwhelm you, and the possible options (responses) might confuse you. A useful approach is to read the stem of the question (the part that asks the question), develop a pool of possible answers drawn from what you already know, then search through the options for the one that most closely matches what is in your pool of answers.

Deciding What to Do When the Right Answer is Not There

- When reading the possible responses to a test question, you might not see your first choice. Since the NCLEX-PN expects you to know the best answer, the responses listed might include your second or third choice. That is why you need a pool of answers from which to draw. Haphazard guessing can be a mistake, because, theoretically, you have only a 25% chance of guessing the correct response to a standard multiple-choice item (although with CAT's selection process you should have a 50% chance of choosing correctly). If, after narrowing down your choices to two and rereading the stem, you still cannot find an answer you want to choose, you must select one and move on. While there is no penalty for guessing, there is a reward in narrowing down the possible responses and choosing from those. And remember, there is a penalty for not choosing an option. No answer is always a wrong answer.

Finding Two Right Answers

- Suppose you've narrowed it down to two responses, and you truly believe both are correct. Before selecting one, reread the stem and be sure you understand exactly what the item is asking. For standard multiple-choice questions, the writers and reviewers planned only one correct answer. Each option is either right or wrong. This type of test item never has more than one correct response.

Debunking the "Pattern"

- Myths about the NCLEX-PN circulate easily and widely. One is that, when in doubt, you should choose answer C. This is not so. There are no pre-established patterns for correct answers. For each item, selecting C without narrowing down your choices will not improve your odds of answering correctly – and it could work against you. Another myth is that if, for example, you miss an endocrine question, you will then get a dozen more like it. This is not so. There is no pattern of content areas. The test items follow the client need-based distribution outlined in the test plan.

Prioritizing the Options

- To answer a question posed in a priority item ("Which action will you take first?"), keep in mind that all four responses represent actions you should take. But you can only choose one, so it must be the one and only action that you should perform first. It might be to meet a physiological need over a psychosocial need, to maintain or establish an airway before attending to breathing and circulation, to ensure a client's safety, to try the least restrictive or invasive method first, to collect data before treating, to address an acute problem rather than a chronic problem, or simply because there is a stepwise protocol that you must follow. When answering a client assignment item, all four clients will need your attention. However, you can only choose one. Select the client who is the least stable or will become much worse if you don't intervene promptly. Using this strategy, you can generally identify the highest priority client.

Using Clinical Reasoning

- If you have never heard of the medication in an item, it might not matter. For example, an item tells you the medication is causing nausea and vomiting. What do you do for any client who is nauseated after taking a medication? Giving medication with food often helps. When in doubt, use your clinical reasoning skills to lead you to the correct response.

Determining What the Question is Asking

- Begin by recognizing who the subject of the question is: the client, the family, or the nurse. Also recognize that the nurse in most questions is actually you. If the question refers to a coworker, you are the one who is delegating to other PNs or to assistive personnel. Then make sure that you understand exactly what the question asks. For example, if it asks which statement requires your intervention, you are looking for something that is wrong, not something that is right.

Avoiding Answer Changing

- In your test-taking experience, you may have changed the correct answer to a wrong answer because you second-guessed yourself. As a competent, entry-level nurse, exercise sound reasoning, but do not underestimate your knowledge and abilities.

Understanding the NCLEX-PN Hospital

- If a supply or piece of equipment is included in an item, consider it available for your use. If a medication is included, expect that it is in the formulary and there is a prescription for it. Also, there is no short staffing in the NCLEX-PN hospital. Nurses always have time to sit at eye level with clients and listen to them.

Tackling Alternate Items

- The majority of test items on the NCLEX-PN appear in the standard, four-option, single-answer, multiple-choice format. There is no set percentage of alternate items. Keep in mind, also, that any item might include multimedia, such as charts, tables, graphics, sound, or video, but you might also see the following specific item formats:
  - o Multiple-response – Selecting one or more correct responses (with no "partial credit")
  - o Fill-in-the-blank – Calculating or measuring a specific quantity correctly
  - o Drag-and-drop – Placing options in the correct order
  - o Hot-spot – Using your mouse to select a correct area within an image
  - o Exhibit – Accessing data from three tabs to help you respond correctly
  - o Audio – Listening to an audio clip with headphones
  - o Graphic options – Selecting the correct option from a group of images

Best Wishes From ATI

- If you have followed a carefully crafted study plan for the NCLEX-PN consistently throughout your nursing program, you will approach the examination equipped for success. All of ATI's NCLEX-preparation tools and products will support you until you meet your ultimate goal of nursing licensure. So, use the materials optimally and go to the testing center with strength and confidence. Success is within your grasp.

- Now, get ready... set... be a practical nurse!

References

National Council of State Boards of Nursing. (2011). NCLEX® Examinations. Chicago, IL: National Council of State Boards of Nursing. Retrieved November 16, 2010, from https://www.ncsbn.org